AMPICILLIN

The Perfect Guide For The Treatment Of Bacterial, Pneumonia And Other Respiratory Tract Infections

Dr. Williams Jones

AMPICILLIN

Ampicillin is a broad-spectrum antibiotic derived from the penicillin family. It is commonly used to treat bacterial infections caused by both Gram-positive and Gram-negative bacteria. It is one of the most widely used antibiotics in the world and has been in use since the early 1960s. Ampicillin is a semisynthetic penicillin, meaning it is produced by the modification of a naturally occurring penicillin molecule. Specifically, it is a beta lactam antibiotic, meaning it has a four-membered ring called a beta lactam, which is essential for its antibacterial activity. It is able to bind to and inhibit enzymes called penicillin binding proteins, which are essential for the production of bacterial cell walls. This prevents the bacteria from growing, thus leading to their destruction. Ampicillin is effective against a wide range of bacterial infections, including infections of the respiratory tract, skin and soft tissue, urinary tract, gastrointestinal tract, and female genital tract. It is also effective against some anaerobic bacteria. It is commonly used to treat bacterial infections such as pneumonia, meningitis, gonorrhea, and salmonellosis. Ampicillin is usually given as an oral or intravenous (IV) dose. It is usually dosed every 8 hours for a period of 5-14 days, depending on the severity and type of infection. It is important to finish the full course of antibiotic therapy, even if symptoms have improved, in order to prevent the development of antibiotic resistance. In addition to its antibiotic properties, ampicillin also has an anti-inflammatory effect, which is useful for treating infections caused by inflammation. It is also used to treat certain types of meningitis, endocarditis, and certain types of sepsis. Ampicillin is generally well-tolerated, though some people may experience side effects such as nausea, vomiting, diarrhea, and skin rash. It is important to tell your doctor if you are pregnant or breastfeeding, as ampicillin may not be suitable in these cases. It is also important to tell your doctor if you are taking any other medications, as ampicillin may interact with some of them. Overall, ampicillin is a safe and effective antibiotic, which is widely used to treat a variety of bacterial infections. It is important to follow the instructions of your doctor, and to finish the full course of antibiotic treatment to ensure the infection is completely cleared.

COMPOSITION AND CHARACTERISTICS OF AMPICILLIN

Ampicillin is a penicillin-based antibiotic that belongs to the aminopenicillin family. It is one of the most widely used antibiotics in the world and has been used to treat a variety of infections for the last fifty years. Ampicillin is an off-white, odorless crystalline powder that is soluble in water and has a molecular weight of 365.4. It has a melting point of around 137°C and a pKa of 2.9. At pH levels of 7.0 or lower, ampicillin is stable and has a relatively long shelf life. Ampicillin is comprised of a beta-lactam ring, which is responsible for its antibiotic activity. This ring is connected to a five-membered thiazolidine ring, and the whole molecule is composed of five nitrogen atoms, three oxygen atoms and one sulfur atom. The beta-lactam ring of ampicillin is responsible for its activity against a variety of bacteria, including Escherichia coli, Staphylococcus aureus, and Pseudomonas acruginosa. Ampicillin works by inhibiting the production of bacterial cell walls. It binds to the bacterial enzyme penicillin-binding protein, which is responsible for the synthesis of peptidoglycan, a component of the bacterial cell wall. By binding to and inhibiting the enzyme, ampicillin prevents the bacteria from producing peptidoglycan, thus preventing the bacteria from replicating. Ampicillin is most commonly used to treat urinary tract infections, sinus infections, and bronchitis. It is also used to treat meningitis, endocarditis, and some types of pneumonia. It is usually administered orally, but can also be given intravenously or intramuscularly. Ampicillin is generally well tolerated, although some side effects may occur. These include nausea, vomiting, diarrhea, and rash. It is important to take the full course of medication prescribed by your doctor to ensure that the infection is completely eliminated. Ampicillin is a penicillin-based antibiotic that is used to treat a variety of infections. It works by preventing the bacteria from replicating by inhibiting the production of bacterial cell walls. It is generally well tolerated, although some side effects can occur. It is important to take the full course of medication prescribed by your doctor to ensure that the infection is completely eliminated.

USES OF AMPICILLIN

Ampicillin is an antibiotic drug commonly used to treat a wide variety of bacterial infections. It belongs to a group of drugs known as penicillins, which are derived from the fungus Penicillium. Ampicillin works by inhibiting the growth of bacteria by interfering with its cell wall formation. This prevents the bacteria from forming new cells and causes them to eventually die. Ampicillin is used to treat many types of bacterial infections, including urinary tract infections, ear infections, sinus infections, and skin infections. It is also used to treat certain sexually transmitted diseases, such as gonorrhea and syphilis. In addition, it can be used to treat infections caused by certain bacteria that are resistant to other antibiotics. Ampicillin is also used to prevent infections in people who are having certain types of surgery. It is also used to prevent recurrent infections in patients who have had a previous infection with a particular type of bacteria. Ampicillin is usually taken orally in the form of a capsule, tablet, or liquid. It is also available as an intravenous (IV) injection or an intramuscular (IM) injection. The dose of ampicillin depends on the type and severity of the infection being treated. It is important to take the medication exactly as prescribed by the doctor. Ampicillin is generally well tolerated by most people, but some may experience side effects, such as nausea, vomiting, diarrhea, or rashes. It is important to contact the doctor immediately if any of these side effects occur. Ampicillin is a safe and effective antibiotic when used as directed by a doctor. It is important to take the medication exactly as prescribed and to complete the entire course of treatment, even if the symptoms of the infection seem to have gone away. This helps to ensure that all of the bacteria causing the infection have been eliminated. Failure to do so can lead to the development of antibiotic-resistant bacteria, which can be difficult to treat. Ampicillin is a commonly used antibiotic drug that is effective in treating a wide variety of bacterial infections. It is generally well tolerated by most people, but side effects can occur. It is important to take the medication exactly as prescribed and to complete the entire course of treatment to ensure that all of the bacteria causing the infection have been eliminated.

SIDE EFFECTS OF AMPICILLIN

Ampicillin is an antibiotic drug that is used to treat bacterial infections such as pneumonia, bronchitis, ear infections, bladder infections, meningitis, and salmonella. While it is generally safe and effective when taken as prescribed, like all antibiotics, it does have some side effects that patients should be aware of. The most common side effects of ampicillin include nausea, vomiting, diarrhea, stomach upset, and abdominal pain. These symptoms are usually mild and should go away after the patient stops taking the drug. In rare cases, a patient may experience an allergic reaction to ampicillin, which can include hives, difficulty breathing, and swelling of the face, lips, tongue, or throat. If any of these symptoms occur, patients should seek immediate medical attention. In addition to gastrointestinal side effects, ampicillin can also cause other side effects. For example, some people may experience headaches, dizziness, or fatigue. Patients may also experience skin rashes, itching, or hives. Some patients may experience an increase in yeast infections while taking ampicillin, which can be uncomfortable and inconvenient. Ampicillin can also cause changes in the body's chemistry, which can lead to serious side effects. For example, some patients may experience an increase in their potassium levels, which can lead to abnormal heart rhythms. Additionally, ampicillin can cause severe liver damage in rare cases. Patients should be aware of the signs of liver damage, including yellowing of the skin or eyes, dark-colored urine, and abdominal pain. If any of these symptoms occur, patients should seek medical attention immediately. Finally, ampicillin can cause anemia, which is an abnormal decrease in red blood cells. Anemia can cause patients to feel weak and tired, and can also lead to other health complications. If a patient has any of these symptoms, they should talk to their doctor about whether ampicillin is the cause. Ampicillin can be a very effective antibiotic when taken as prescribed, but it does have some potential side effects. Patients should be aware of the potential side effects, and contact their doctor if any of these symptoms occur. Additionally, patients should be aware of the signs of serious side effects, including yellowing of the skin or eyes, dark-colored urine, or abdominal pain. If any of these symptoms occur, patients should seek immediate medical attention.

PRECAUTIONS OF AMPICILLIN

Ampicillin is an antibiotic used to treat a variety of bacterial infections. It is a member of the penicillin family and works by inhibiting the growth of bacteria. Although ampicillin can be effective in treating bacterial infections, there are some precautions that should be taken into consideration when using this medication. The first precaution when taking ampicillin is to be aware of possible allergies. People with allergies to penicillin or cephalosporin antibiotics should not take ampicillin. Additionally, if you are taking any other medications, it is important to discuss these with your doctor before starting ampicillin as there may be drug interactions. The second precaution when taking ampicillin is to be aware of potential side effects. Common side effects of ampicillin include nausea, vomiting, diarrhea, and abdominal pain. In rare cases, more serious side effects such as severe allergic reactions, seizures, and kidney toxicity have been reported. If you experience any of these side effects, contact your doctor right away. The third precaution is to monitor for signs of an overgrowth of bacteria. Ampicillin can disrupt the natural balance of bacteria in your body, leading to an overgrowth of certain bacteria. This can cause infections such as thrush and urinary tract infections. If you experience any unusual symptoms, contact your doctor right away. The fourth precaution is to avoid taking ampicillin for longer than necessary. Long-term use of ampicillin can lead to antibiotic resistance, meaning that the medication will no longer be effective in treating the infection. Additionally, prolonged use of ampicillin can lead to an imbalance of bacteria in the body, leading to potential health complications. The fifth precaution when taking ampicillin is to be aware of potential drug interactions. Ampicillin can interact with other medications, such as anticoagulants, nonsteroidal anti-inflammatory drugs, and oral contraceptives. If you are taking any other medications, it is important to discuss these with your doctor before starting ampicillin. Finally, it is essential to take ampicillin as directed by your doctor. Ampicillin should be taken exactly as prescribed and should not be taken in larger or smaller amounts than recommended. Additionally, do not stop taking ampicillin without consulting your doctor. Ampicillin can be an effective antibiotic for treating bacterial infections. However, it is important to take precautions in order to reduce the risk of side effects and potential interactions. Be sure to discuss any allergies or other medications with your doctor and follow their instructions carefully when taking ampicillin.

INTERACTIONS

Ampicillin is a β-lactam antibiotic used to treat a wide range of bacterial infections. It is a semi-synthetic derivative of penicillin, derived from the soil bacterium called Penicillium. It was first discovered in 1956 and was the first penicillin that could be used to treat infections caused by gram-negative bacteria. Ampicillin is effective against a wide range of bacteria, including both gram-positive and gram-negative bacteria. It is also able to penetrate the outer membrane of gram-negative bacteria, which makes it especially effective against these types of bacteria. Ampicillin works by inhibiting the synthesis of bacterial cell walls. This occurs through the binding of the ampicillin molecule to the enzyme transpeptidase, which is responsible for the cross-linking of peptidoglycan molecules in the bacterial cell wall. By binding to transpeptidase, ampicillin prevents the formation of peptidoglycan, which is an essential component of the bacterial cell wall. The lack of peptidoglycan leads to a weakening of the cell wall which then causes the cell to rupture and die. Ampicillin is also known to interact with other antibiotics, such as tetracycline and chloramphenicol. The interaction between ampicillin and tetracycline is known as synergism, where the two antibiotics act together to inhibit bacterial growth more effectively than either one alone. This is because ampicillin binds to transpeptidase, preventing the formation of peptidoglycan, while tetracycline inhibits the synthesis of proteins that are essential for bacterial growth. On the other hand, the interaction between ampicillin and chloramphenicol is known as antagonism, where one of the antibiotics reduces the effectiveness of the other. This is because chloramphenicol binds to an enzyme involved in protein synthesis, while ampicillin binds to transpeptidase, preventing the formation of peptidoglycan. Ampicillin is also known to interact with mammalian cells. It binds to the penicillin binding proteins (PBPs) found in mammalian cells and disrupts the cell membrane. This leads to cell death, which can be beneficial for the treatment of certain infections, such as meningitis. However, this can also lead to toxic effects, such as kidney failure, if the dosage is too high or if it is given for too long. In addition to its interactions with other antibiotics and mammalian cells, ampicillin can also interact with human enzymes. Ampicillin is known to inhibit the enzyme β-lactamase, which is responsible for the breakdown of β-lactam antibiotics, such as penicillin. Therefore, when ampicillin is combined with other β-lactam antibiotics, it can increase the effectiveness of the other antibiotics by preventing their breakdown by β-lactamase. Overall, ampicillin is a widely used antibiotic that has a variety of interactions that can be beneficial or detrimental, depending on the situation. It is important to understand the interactions of ampicillin in order to use it safely and effectively.

DOSAGE

Ampicillin is an antibiotic medication used to treat a variety of bacterial infections. It belongs to the penicillin group of drugs and is normally prescribed to treat respiratory, urinary tract, gastrointestinal, and skin infections. It works by stopping the growth of bacteria. Ampicillin is usually taken orally in the form of tablets, capsules, or a liquid suspension. The dose of ampicillin depends on the type and severity of infection being treated. It is important to take ampicillin exactly as prescribed by your doctor. Do not take more or less than the amount recommended.

The usual adult dose of ampicillin for mild to moderate infections is 250 to 500 milligrams (mg) every 6 to 8 hours, or 500 to 875 mg every 12 hours. For more severe infections, the dose may be increased to 1000 mg every 6 to 8 hours. For children, the dosage is based on their weight and the severity of the infection. For infants under 3 months of age, the usual dose is 25 to 50 mg per kilogram (kg) of body weight every 12 hours. For older children and adolescents, the usual dose is 50 to 100 mg per kg of body weight every 6 to 12 hours. In some cases, a healthcare provider may prescribe a one-time dose of ampicillin. This is usually done to treat severe infections that require a larger dose of the medication. The usual one-time dose for adults is 2 grams (g). For children, the dose is based on their weight. Ampicillin is usually taken until the infection has cleared up. This may take several days or even weeks. It is important to complete the full course of treatment, even if you start to feel better after a few days. Stopping the medication too soon may cause the infection to come back. It is important to take ampicillin exactly as prescribed. Do not take more or less than the recommended dose. Do not stop taking it or change the dosage without first talking to your doctor. If you miss a dose, take it as soon as you remember. If it is close to the time for your next dose, skip the missed dose and take the next one as usual. Do not take two doses at the same time. Ampicillin can cause side effects such as nausea, vomiting, diarrhea, and skin rash. If these occur, contact your doctor. Tell your doctor if you are pregnant or breastfeeding before taking ampicillin. The dosage of ampicillin depends on the type and severity of the infection being treated, as well as the age and weight of the patient. It is important to take ampicillin exactly as prescribed and not to stop taking it or change the dosage without first talking to your doctor. Side effects such as nausea, vomiting, diarrhea, and skin rash may occur. If these occur, contact your doctor.

STORAGE

Ampicillin is an antibiotic that belongs to a group of drugs called penicillins. It is used to treat a wide variety of bacterial infections, such as urinary tract infections, ear infections, skin infections, and respiratory infections. It is also used to prevent certain types of bacterial infections in people who are undergoing certain types of medical procedures. The storage of ampicillin is important for its effectiveness and safety. Ampicillin should be stored at room temperature, away from light and moisture. It should not be stored in the bathroom or near a sink. Other medications should be stored separately from ampicillin and the storage area should be kept clean and organized. Ampicillin should be stored in its original container, with the lid tightly closed. It should not be exposed to direct sunlight or excessive heat. If the original container is not available, ampicillin can be stored in a light-resistant, airtight container. The expiration date should be checked before taking the medication, and any medication that has expired should be discarded. Ampicillin should not be frozen, as this could damage the drug and make it less effective. It should also not be mixed with other medications or solutions, as this could result in a dangerous reaction. If ampicillin needs to be taken with other medications, it should be taken at least one hour before or two hours after the other medications. Ampicillin should be kept out of reach of children and pets. It should not be taken by anyone other than the person it was prescribed for. If the medication is no longer needed, it should be disposed of properly. Any unused or expired ampicillin should be returned to the pharmacy for proper disposal. Ampicillin should be stored at room temperature, away from light and moisture. It should be stored in its original container, with the lid tightly closed. It should not be frozen or mixed with other medications or solutions. It should also be kept out of reach of children and pets. If the medication is no longer needed, it should be disposed of properly.

CONCLUSION

Ampicillin is a type of antibiotic used to treat a variety of bacterial infections. It is effective against a wide range of gram-positive and gram-negative bacteria, including some of the more serious infections such as endocarditis, meningitis, and pneumonia. It is generally well-tolerated and has few side effects. In conclusion, ampicillin is a useful antibiotic with a broad range of applications.

It is effective against a range of bacterial infections, including some of the more serious ones. It is generally well-tolerated and has few side effects. As with any medication, it is important to be aware of the potential side effects and consult a doctor if any occur. Additionally, it is important to use ampicillin as directed and to not overuse it or use it to treat infections that it is not intended to treat. With proper use and monitoring, ampicillin can be an effective tool to treat bacterial infections.

Made in the USA
Coppell, TX
17 March 2024

30213780R00022